Does Hypnosis *Really* Work?

Bill Duffy, CHt

First printing March 2012
Second printing July 2012

ISBN: 978-0-9858766-0-9

Cover design: Mary Francis Hanson
Front cover images: Shotas/Dreamstime.com

Printed by:
Grelin Press, P.O. Box 367
New Kensington, PA 15068
Tel: (724) 334-8240   grelinpress@aol.com
www.grelinpress.com

To my wife, Mary, for her patience during the lonely hours she spent while I was at my computer and to my niece, Mary Francis Hanson, whose creative abilities helped to give this book a professional look.

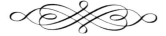

CONTENTS

INTRODUCTION

DOES HYPNOSIS *REALLY* WORK ?

If I'm asked that question again, it will be for the 330th time since I hypnotized my first subject in 1945. I'm really not sure about that number, but I really don't think it's an exaggeration. In fact, I'm really surprised when that question isn't asked before I begin a hypnotic session.

Can't say that I blame you or anyone for a lack of knowledge about hypnosis. You can't be expected to realize that hypnosis can be of help in eliminating personal problems such as smoking, obesity, anxiety or one of many other unwanted behaviors. We hypnotists have done a very poor job of educating the public and the medical profession about the role that hypnosis can play in implementing the treatment of these human behaviors.

The only exposure that some relatively few people have had to hypnosis is the result of their attendance at a performance by a stage hypnotist. These performances are intended to entertain and certainly don't show hypnosis in its more valued role of helping a person's health or quality of life. It must be acknowledged, however, that stage hypnosis has surely helped to keep the public aware of it when interest in it was waning.

I was completely ignorant of the place or merits of hypnosis when I attended my psychology class during my Junior year at Duquesne University. This all changed remarkably during a lecture by my professor Doctor A. Lester Pierce. He began the lecture by stating that we had a very mysterious, yet very capable, subconscious mind and was going to prove it to us.

Taking a volunteer from the class, he hypnotized him and proceeded to give him what he termed a "post-hypnotic" suggestion. He said, "I'm going to awaken you and I'm going to the front of the class. When I tear the newspaper on my desk, you're going to experience a pain in your stomach ... not one that will hurt your system but you will feel it. You're not going to remember this suggestion consciously—but your subconscious mind will."

Pierce awakened him and the eye-blinking young man said, "That was very relaxing." Was this really going to work? This so-called post-hypnotic suggestion? After about five minutes, the professor, in the middle of a sentence, picked up the newspaper and tore it slowly. We all stared at the boy as he got this strange look on his face. He jumped from his seat, grabbed his stomach and yelled, "Ouch!" And added, "Why did I do that?" He sat down again. That wasn't the end of the demonstration. Five minutes later, the professor picked up the newspaper and tore it again. Same reaction.

The professor then went to the boy's seat, said, "Look at me." When the boy did, Professor Pierce said. "When I count to three, the suggestion I gave your subconscious mind concerning the newspaper will be erased. One, two, three." He went to the front of the room, picked up the newspaper and tore it. No reaction.

I was hooked. I couldn't wait to learn how to perform this seemingly magic and astounding thing that the professor had demonstrated. Nagging at him, he finally agreed to teach me. Before I graduated the following year and joined military service, I thought I was an accomplished hypnotist. I wasn't and professor Pierce made me promise to seek additional training before hypnotizing any subjects.

I didn't keep my promise. Stationed in the Philippines, I hypnotized a friend who complained of being very homesick. To my surprise, he went into a deep trance. I had him flying over his house, seeing his mother standing in his back yard.

It was my own personal proof that I could hypnotize a subject into a deep trance.

But I did study and train for almost five years after returning from service. A medical hypnotist who had worked in military hospitals was my teacher.

Does hypnosis really work? My practice for these many years has proved countless times that it does.

I'd like to tell you why and how.

1

WHO STARTED THIS
HYPNOSIS BUSINESS ANYHOW?

Only the Good Lord knows.

All cultures and civilizations seem to have had a part in a practice whereby one human being had been able to exercise a personal influence over another. Suffice it to say that, from the savages who dwelled in caves, the ancient Persians and Jews, the African races, the Orient nations, the Egyptian Gnostics and the early church, all practiced some form by which they could affect the thoughts and actions of others.

Universal attention was drawn to a so-called animal magnetism by a Viennese doctor, Franz Anton Mesmer, who was born in 1734. He used magnets to put a person into a spell, treating and curing many types of disease.

Although scoffed by many in his profession, he was moderately successful in his endeavors. Mesmer left Austria after the practice of animal magnetism was banned. Going to France, he found many adherents as well as opponents to his methods. In Germany, his methods met with better reception. Magnetism was introduced into hospital treatment and flourished so much that after Mesmer's death in 1815, a monument was placed on his grave as a tribute to his work.

Literally, hundreds of physicians began practicing various forms of Mesmer's original principles. Without some form of chemical anesthetic available, they used suggestion to put patients into a trance state, allowing them to perform surgical operations and cure many diseases.

One of the most remarkable cases of this type was the works of a Doctor James Esdaile, a Scottish surgeon who began practicing in India. He performed over a thousand surgical operations with hypnosis, no anesthetic— none available. Included in these operations were about 20 amputations. No anesthetic. None available.

What happened? Why doesn't the medical profession use improved methods of hypnosis to perform operations without anesthetic? There are some very rare cases where such operations are performed, but not many. What happened was, in 1838, ether was "discovered" and introduced to the medical profession ... that's what happened. Goodbye hypnosis. Too time consuming. In fact, medical professionals turned up their collective noses to hypnotism and it went into disfavor universally.

Thanks to relatively few believers who continued to practice hypnosis, and the performers who earned a living by hypnotizing people on the stage, hypnosis stayed alive. Through the ensuing years, hypnosis had many good days and many bad days.

I can vividly remember the 1960s. Hypnosis had started to gain some recognition as a therapeutic tool and I felt a little more comfortable when I acknowledged that I was a hypnotist. But some friends still thought I was dealing in the paranormal. I had problems connecting with anyone in the medical profession. Once, I was asked to leave a doctor's office. I wonder what that doctor might think today since he knows now that the American and British Medical Associations approve of the use of hypnosis as a therapeutic tool.

Today, a goodly number of my referrals come from doctors.

In fact, the first doctor I received a referral from called and said, "Anyone who can get my wife to quit smoking must be performing some kind of magic. I'd like to talk to you." Unaware that her husband was a doctor, I had hypnotized a woman to become a non-smoker. She quit after two sessions.

This happened quite early in my practice. Ever since my first meeting with her doctor husband, a DO, I've been receiving referrals from him to work with many of his patients. In years following, other doctors have also referred their patients for hypnosis.

2

FIRST OF ALL, WHAT IS HYPNOSIS?

Webster defines hypnosis as a "state that resembles sleep but is induced by a person whose suggestions are readily accepted by the subject." The word hypnosis comes from the Greek *hypnos* (or sleep), a name given to the procedure by an English doctor, James Braid, who used suggestion to induce a feeling of deep relaxation.

Braid stated that, "Hypnosis is a state of physical relaxation accompanied by and induced by mental concentration."

I often begin lectures by explaining what I feel is the difference in hypnosis and sleep. I point out that when people went to bed last night, their conscious and subconscious minds traded places and their conscious mind, in effect, turned over and went to sleep. Their subconscious minds, as they always have, stayed busy running their autonomous systems. As this mind has

17

since the moment they were born, it continued to run all those important functions such as their hearts, their respiration and the organs of their body that kept them perking.

"When you sleep," I point out, "you probably also have dreams, but you may not remember some of them, depending on how deeply asleep you were when the dreams occurred. But dreaming is sometimes just musing on the part of the subconscious. Or, this unusual mind could be trying to give you a message— generally in a symbolic manner.

"When you're hypnotized, much the same thing happens, with one difference. Although your two minds change places, under hypnosis your conscious mind goes into a very relaxed mode, but it does not go to sleep. It stays alert and hears everything the hypnotist says. The subconscious mind also hears and, for reasons I'll explain later, accepts suggestions of a positive nature. Because of the innate characteristics of the sub-conscious mind, these suggestions are exceedingly more effective than similar suggestions a person might give to their conscious mind."

Most hypnotists will tell you that all hypnosis is really self-hypnosis. They mean that all you do as the hypnotist talks to you is hear the suggestions and either accept or reject them. Accepting the suggestions to relax, for example, you relax your body and mind, and go into a dream-like state called hypnosis. It's a very, pleasant feeling when you're hypnotized. A woman once related that she felt like "a damp dishrag" while she was in the deep hypnosis.

While a hypnotized person is in this very relaxed state, the hypnotist can establish a connection with their subconscious mind and offer suggestions which affect conscious decisions, eliminate unwanted behavior patterns and fears, manage pain or probe for the reason for a specified problem.

So again, the definition of hypnosis. Hypnosis is an altered state of consciousness which resembles sleep, but is not sleep, a state of deep relaxation during which the subject has an increased response to proper suggestions given to their subconscious mind.

In effect, suggestions given under hypnosis are post-hypnotic. For example, the suggestions given to a subject while in a trance state are meant to help the subject after he or she is awake. An obese subject, for example, receives positive suggestions to increase determination, control eating habits and have sufficient incentive to achieve the desired results in daily practice.

There are two basic types of hypnosis; *Hetero-hypnosis,* when a hypnotist offers suggestions to a subject; and *self-hypnosis* when a person becomes both hypnotist and subject, offering suggestions to his or her own subconscious mind.

3

SOME QUESTIONS AND ANSWERS

Here's my answer to many of the questions I'm asked about hypnosis:

Who can be hypnotized?   Probably you. Most people will reach a pleasant state of relaxation . . . which will produce a light trance, a state where many suggestions to the subconscious mind will be surprisingly effective. Most people I hypnotize for smoking cessation, weight reduction and other similar behavior patterns need only be in a light trance to achieve positive results.

Naturally, there are exceptions. Mentally disadvantaged persons. Generally, those people who cannot keep a positive concentration level will be distracted and not respond. I've had some level of success with

Alzheimer patients, but the effect of suggestions seems to erode after a relatively short time.

Rarely a person may be hypnotized so easily that it poses a problem for them. The networks do not show a hypnotist actually inducing a trance for obvious reasons. There are relatively few people who will go into a hypnotic trance with only a simple few words of suggestion.

Many years ago I met a woman who was an "immediate" subject. Anyone, even someone who wasn't a hypnotist could put "Helen" into a trace with the mere words, "Sleep, Helen." Fortunately I was able to help her. Under hypnosis, I gave her the suggestion that, unless she said aloud, "I want to be hypnotized," she would not be. Her subconscious was given a block against going into a trance unless she agreed.

It doesn't mean you have a weak mind if you can be hypnotized. It takes an average mind with normal creative ability to be a good subject. Even if you're a brilliant scientist with a whooping big IQ, you can be hypnotized. So, regardless which category fits you, you'd be a darn good subject.

It's always amusing when some men, usually an engineer or someone who deals with figures or scientific data comes to be hypnotized. They are quick to assure me, "I really don't think I can be hypnotized, but ..." But it's no surprise when they become very deep trance subjects.

An associate of mine in my marketing office, approached me one morning. She said, "I understand that you're a hypnotist." "Yes, I am," I replied, expecting some negative reaction from her. "Interesting," she said. "What's that all about?"

After giving her my ten-cent speech about what hypnosis is and how it works, She said the expected. "I doubt if I can be hypnotized."

Maybe, I thought, she was right. This woman had an IQ that was out of sight. She was respected all over town as a "brain." She rarely smiled. She scared me.

"I want you to try," she said and it almost sounded like a dare. But I tried and to my surprise, it only took about a minute and she was in what I felt was a medium trance. Was she hypnotized? Only one way to be sure....

"In just a moment," I told her, "I'm going to awaken you. Since you have a meeting scheduled in about a half hour, you're going to have to go to the front door in the reception room. When you touch the front door knob, you will get very sleepy and stop. You will go to the couch and sit down and immediately fall asleep. Your conscious mind is not going to remember this suggestion, but your subconscious mind will and it will happen." I repeated this suggestion twice more and awakened her. She smiled weakly and said, "That was very relaxing. But, as I said, I don't think I was hypnotized."

I made my excuses and followed her out to the reception room. Touching the front door knob, she paused and went to the couch. "For some reason," she said, "I'm very sleepy," then went to the couch and fell asleep.

I had to be sure to erase the post-hypnotic suggestion. Would she get sleepy the next time she touched the door knob? She probably would. Better safe than sorry. I went to the couch, said her name and awakened her. "Look at me," I said. "The suggestion I gave about the front door knob is erased. One, two. three."

What does it feel like to be hypnotized? As evidenced by what you've already read, hypnosis is a very relaxed state, feeling just like that one woman described, "a damp dishrag." How deep a dream-like state you reach depends as much on you as on the hypnotist. Almost everyone who is hypnotized reports that it is a wonderful feeling of relaxation. "I felt like I was floating …" "I found myself in a place of peace and quiet…" "What a wonderful pleasantly heavy feeling …" "It seemed like it was only minutes since you started talking to me …" "I heard everything you said."

Some people feel as though they weren't hypnotized. Giving them a post-hypnotic suggestion convinces them. It's a rare case when a person isn't able to relax to the depth where positive suggestions are effective.

Some years ago, a man got very irritated when I told him that he wouldn't be able to remember the number six when I asked him to count from one to ten. "That's the damnest, foolishest thing I've ever heard," he said when I awakened him. "First of all, I wasn't hypnotized. I heard everything you said." I had purposely told his conscious mind that he would remember about the numbers, but he still wouldn't remember six.

He rose from the easy chair and started out of the room. "Wait a minute," I said. "Count to ten for me."

"Phooey," he said, "that'll never happen." "Humor me," I urged him. He stopped, glared at me and started counting. He couldn't remember the number six. Guess what he said then!

You really don't feel too much different when you're in a hypnotic state.

But you get the idea. It's a great and relaxing feeling!

Are there any dangers? No. You don't surrender your mind to the hypnotist. And if you don't want to be hypnotized, you shouldn't be seeing the hypnotist in the first place. But if you are seeking help, please make sure that he or she is certified. There are many organizations that certify their members under strict guidelines. The National Guild of Hypnotists, an international organization of about 55,000 members, is one such organization. As a member of NGH and the Hypnotism Society of Pennsylvania. I have met strict requirements to be certified by both groups.

Can there be any problems? Not any more than there would be with a psychiatrist, psychologist, clinician or any other professional treating a person for one of the many human behavioral problems. Still, and I know it will sound very opinionated, but I think there aren't any problems when you are hypnotized by a qualified hypnotist. With hypnosis, anything done can be undone … anything undone can be restored. That's not always the case with many licensed professionals.

What if the hypnotist leaves while you're in a trance? This is a question asked every time I teach a class. If you're in a trance and the hypnotist decides to leave the room and doesn't return for an extended period of time, you'll just awaken and wonder where he or she went. No one will stay in a trance for very long if left unattended.

Any special talents needed to be a hypnotist? Absolutely not. Perhaps a desire to help people. Having an innate talent for understanding their motivations and problems also helps. It does take a lot of dedication ... plus study and experience ... to offer the best to those who can benefit from effective hypnosis counseling.

What are the areas where hypnosis can help?   When I try to answer this question and list the areas where hypnosis can help a fellow human being, my answer usually seems ridiculous to most. That's because there are a very few behavioral and physiological problems which can't be helped with hypnosis. Not "all of the time with all of the people, but most of the time with most of the people."   Plus one other very important condition of the person's mind. *He or she has to want to be helped.*

During a class, when I hand out a paper listing the problems and areas where hypnosis can be of help, members of the class read the list and look at me with an obvious look of disbelief on their faces.

"Really," one man remarked, "looks like you've listed almost every problem a person can have."

He's just about right

This is my list and I'll bet I've forgotten a few:

Stress and anxiety	Phobias & Fears	Stuttering
Smoking Cessation	Weight Reduction	Allergies
Thumb Sucking	Bed Wetting	Obstetrics
Pain Management	Symptom Removal	Surgery
Drug Addiction	Nail Biting	Insomnia
Alcohol Addiction	Sexual Abuse	Healing
Talent Enhancement	Impotence	Sports
Motivation	Dentistry	Memory

… and others which may have to do with a person's behavior or mental and physical well-being

4

OLD HABITS DIE HARD

Some scientists insist that many of us have an inborn tendency toward developing specific habit patterns. In other words, we genetically may be headed toward being a grumpy old person. Can't say I totally disagree. I know a guy who **had** to be born that way.

It usually doesn't work just like that. Habits, good or bad, can be created by our environment, our relationships and our own hand but they don't become habits until we work on them—and practice! Then they find their way into our subconscious minds because we have created a pathway for them and they become ingrained— a habit that we are not even aware of doing or saying— often just a reaction to a specified set of circumstances.

Those who grind their teeth or bite their nails are sometimes aware of the habit but many times not. A fear of the dark which was created at an early age after watching a scary movie continues as a reaction through life, even though logic dictates otherwise. There are a limitless number of habits which are both good and unwanted. Do you know someone who is constantly interrupting others as they talk? How about the person who always goes you one better when you relate a story?

Good habits also have been created by a pathway well traveled. Patience is a virtue but it takes practice to develop it. If you are a patient person, you may have had to bite your tongue a few times before the habit established a pathway and became a permanent part of your life style.

Many bad habits are created because we associate them with other actions we desire. A person states they smoke because it helps relax them; a person snacks because it takes their minds off their problems, a person bites their nails because it relieves nervous tension—all totally because it makes them feel good. It becomes a compulsion which they usually cannot consciously control.

Bad habits are easy targets for hypnotic suggestions. As long as persons want to rid themselves of undesirable habits, hypnosis will do the job. These suggestions "unpave" the pathway and resurface it with a new habit pattern.

Many years ago, a subject asked for help with breaking, what she considered a "terrible" habit. She all too frequently corrected her friends, even about the most unimportant facts. If a friend said it was 42 degrees outside, she would correct her and say, "No, I heard it was 44 degrees." If her friend said it was time the high school football team won a game, she would say, "But they did win three weeks ago." She was forever putting in her "two cents worth." It didn't seem to matter if someone's statement was true or false, she had to make a contrary remark. She was embarrassed every time, but she was never able to catch herself in time to keep her mouth shut.

Fortunately, she didn't try to correct me when I told her that she was feeling very sleepy although she probably wanted to!

She was a good subject, and the suggestions given her were obvious. I simply told her that she would bite her tongue—literally—every time she had the urge to add a comment to a friend's statement. When she raised an eyebrow when I made that suggestion, I hastened to add, "Not hard, but a gentle bite—just enough for you to recognize you should smile and say nothing." And because "biting one's tongue" is a universally accepted symbol for keeping quiet when you shouldn't talk, it was the perfect suggestion for the occasion.

Subject called two weeks later and stated, "I bit my tongue five times that first week and just once so far this week!"

5

HOW HYPNOSIS CAN HELP

Remember, behavioral problems may have their roots in past environments, genetics or other physiological or purely medical conditions. Before seeking help from a hypnotist, it is recommended you check with your doctor.

Here's how hypnosis can help some of these more common problems:

Weight Control. Hypnosis allows you to take control of your eating habits and weaken the cravings for those foods which create your weight problem. Combined with a proper exercise regimen, your new program of control will achieve the desired result. Hypnosis helps you to reduce your mealtime intake, eliminate eating between meals and, very important to a successful program, help you not eat within a few hours before going to bed. *Nothing is worse than taking food to bed with you!*

There often are psychological problems underlying the reasons for uncontrolled eating habits and, as suggested previously, professional advice should be obtained. Many person's genetic background also can contribute to obesity. And there are those people who simply eat too much, eat the wrong food and eat at the wrong time.

Obesity, evidently, does seem to "run in the family," often because members of a given family have bone structures which can support more body mass. The weight problem occurs more frequently with them than with a person of slight build.

Weight loss, then, becomes a relative equation. Hypnosis helps to set goals which are realistic. The heavier person and the slight-built subject should set the loss of different poundage as goals. A woman I hypnotized for weight loss weighed 270 pounds when we had our first session. Asked what she wanted to lose through hypnosis, she said, "I want to get down to 150 pounds." I told her that was unrealistic and she should set a more reasonable goal. She was disappointed, but agreed when I suggested we set a first goal of 220 pounds. A slightly built woman of 170 easily reached her goal of 145 pounds. Actually, both these women lost about the same percentage of pounds. The first woman was satisfied when additional sessions helped her to get down to 185 pounds. Her large frame seemed to carry this weight comfortably.

Oddly enough, almost identical suggestions were used with both these women.

Smoking Cessation. One reason that hypnosis for smoking cessation doesn't work for most people in a group audience is that people want to quit smoking for different reasons. Person "A" may have a bad heart. Person "B" may have poor circulation. Person "C" may have shortness of breath. And what about the mother or father who wants to stop smoking because they don't want their children to pick up the habit?

Smoking is both a chemical and personal habit problem. Nicotine from cigarette smoke enters the blood stream and creates a level of the drug which the smoker continues to maintain and feels comfortable with. When a smoker doesn't have a cigarette for an extended period of time, a craving rears up. The patch, chewing gum and other nicotine producing aids help. But they don't help with the real problem which smokers have when they want to quit smoking.

The habit patterns a smoker builds up through years of smoking are very difficult to break. A cigarette with morning coffee. While talking on the phone. A mid-morning fix. Eating a snack just so a cigarette will taste good. After each meal. That last cigarette before going to bed. Others too, depending on the smoker's life style.

After years of hypnotizing people to help them break the smoking habit, this daily pattern of smoking is the real monster. The suggestions I give are, first, to reinforce the desire to quit smoking—the reasons why they need to quit; second, to distract them from the craving by the substitution of thoughts or actions that bypass the craving.

These suggestions are put into the subconscious mind. The smoker can break the habit if he or she works with them. The first few days after a hypnotic session are the important days. The effectiveness of suggestions grow when they are followed; if a smoker refuses to work with them suggestions lose their strength and the habit returns. It is important to remember that nicotine isn't the major problem—long after nicotine cravings are out of the picture, the habit pattern can still exist—and hypnosis and the subconscious mind are the answers to breaking the *habit* of smoking.

Anxiety. It seems that Americans are a bunch of "worry-warts." Everywhere you turn you meet someone who insist they have anxiety attacks. Worrying about school, work, the family budget, relationships, and anything which interferes with their peace of mind.

A little bit of worry is a good thing. It serves a useful purpose because it prepares us for life's problems. But unnecessary worry does interfere with not only peace of mind, it prevents one from leading a normal life, leads to anxiety attacks and disturbs not only our own life but also the lives of those around us.

Case in point. A woman of 38 who worried incessantly about her boss' appraisal of her work. She reported that she had received excellent reports from district managers on her work. She was always on time for work and spent many hours after regular work hours correcting reports prepared by fellow workers she supervised. In spite of her work ethic and periodic praise by her boss, she spent many hours fretting about whether he appreciated her devotion and attention to her job. No reason in the world why she should have had anxiety attacks.

Essence of suggestions given her when hypnotized: Her worries were an exaggeration of the actual facts. She had no logical reasons for her concern over her boss' evaluation of her work. Even though he might not often express his satisfaction, other evidence proved his appreciation. Every report from fellow workers verified her excellent work ethic.

Action suggested to her subconscious mind: Every day, for ten minutes before she went to work, she was to meditate on the excellent work substantiated by praise of fellow workers and her boss. This meditative state would convince her of the validity of this acceptance and make her proud. This pride would stay with her through the day and lessen her worry about the job. Each day this meditation would increase her assurance that she was doing an excellent job. She would be worry-free and free of anxiety about her job. She would enjoy her work every day and look forward to going to the office.

Another case. A teacher at a local elementary school, was anxious that she was disliked by her home room class. She worried to the point where it affected her relationships with her own two children and her husband.

She admitted in our initial session that she couldn't identify specific reasons for her concerns, but said "I have this pervasive feeling that these eight and nine year olds don't like me. They can't wait to leave the class-room."

In addition to her home room duties, she taught the class mathematics. It was during these math teaching sessions that she had her negative feelings. Questioning didn't uncover any substantial reasons for her feelings. She refused my suggestion that she ask the school principal if he had received any negative comments from parents. We discussed specifics of math lessons and acknowledged that this was the first real exposure that her students had to rather complicated math problems. She admitted that some students were having difficulty understanding multiplication problems.

Second session. Subject was difficult to relax but finally went into a fairly deep trance. I awakened her and explained the details of the type of suggestions I was going to give her. Then I hypnotized her again.

Points I made to her subconscious mind: She had no concrete evidence to support her negative feelings. She had to be aware that math was a subject requiring serious concentration by her students—and she had to emphasize with her students about this difficulty and assure them that it would come to them. (She gave me the impression that she didn't have a "personal touch.") She needed to use a hands-on connection with individual students. Walk down the aisles and give individual attention to those needing it. Assure them that their brothers, sisters and/or friends had the same difficulty at first but they were now doing all kinds of math problems. I told her to learn to help her students to relax and relax herself—to smile—praise a student who correctly worked a problem—enjoy what she was doing. (*Repeat essence of preceding suggestions*)

Third session. (She revealed that she rarely spoke about her math class at home with her husband or two daughters) Suggested she do so at the dinner table— not to air her concerns but just to discuss some of the math problems the class was working on. She would find that by talking about the class she would feel more and more relaxed as she got feedback from her family. I reminded her that her daughters had experienced learning basic math too.

(*Then repeated essence of verbalisms given during second session.*)

I then concentrated on her mental approach. "When you awaken on a school day morning, you arise with a pleasant feeling that the day allows another opportunity to help children learn. You look forward to walking into the classroom. You walk in with a smile and greet each child as they enter with a cheerful greeting. You're going to learn each child's first name and address them with it. If you don't know their first names, get name tags and have them wear them until you do. When you put a problem on the board, explain it and then walk up and down the aisles, helping where you can and calling each child by his or her first name. At this point, if you don't know their first name, ask and use it The children will respond, and so will you, to a more personal touch. Make learning fun—for you and the children. If you can relate a story about one of your daughter's math experiences, all the better.

"And you'll find you will have a pleasant and wonderful feeling of relaxation. And a great feeling of accomplishment. Feel this relaxation on the way home and during the evening. Tell your family about your day at school. And when you brush your teeth before bedtime, look in the mirror. Good day, wasn't it? Tomorrow will be too!"

I'm not in the habit of trying to help someone do their job, but in the case of this teacher, her anxiety problem was more the result of her relationships with her students than anything else.

Fears and Phobias. There are fears born out of respect for certain situations we face: fear of flying, high spaces, snakes, some animals, for example. I consider them as rational fears and they are shared by many. Even so, I've had success helping people overcome these fears with hypnosis, usually in two or three sessions.

When a fear gets out of proportion to reality, a phobia is created.

A friend of mine was so fearful of flying that he couldn't watch movies that showed the actors flying in regular scheduled aircraft. He trembled when he thought that his boss might ask him to fly to a distant branch office. He realized that his refusal could cost him his job.

One day about noon, he walked into my office. He looked pale and stammered as he said, "I have to fly this afternoon. My mother is dying. As you know, she lives in St. Louis. I gotta go. I gotta fly. You have to hypnotize me."

Because of his nervousness he was difficult to relax. Finally, he sighed and slowly sank into a comfortable relaxed state. My suggestions to his subconscious mind were somewhat different because I knew him so well. I told him he was being a dumb wit because he feared flying. "You know as well as I do that statistics prove that flying in a well-maintained, modern jet will be a safer way to get to St. Louis than driving there. When you fly there today, you'll be one of thousands of people taking off and landing at one of the hundreds of airports in this country. Arriving safely, you hear?" I repeated this same suggestion several times.

"Now relax, man. These facts you just heard land deep in your subconscious mind and they start right now to lessen more and more each minute the irrational fear you have of flying. Nothing to it, you'll love the wonderful feeling of being in the air, safely on your way to see your mom.

"Let me show you. You can see yourself now. You've given your ticket at the gate. You're getting off the ramp into the plane. Smiling faces at the door. Lots of people inside, putting their carry-on luggage in the ports above. It's amazing how calm you are. In your seat, you watch the plane taxi then take off. Great feeling of comfort and safety. You arrive in St. Louis. You smile and feel very relaxed. Nothing to it, was there?" I paused. "Call me after you see your mom."

He didn't call for about a week. "Sorry to say," he reported, "my mother died the morning after I get there. I just got back yesterday." I could sense his smile over the phone. "How could I have been so afraid of flying!"

Those with phobias must confront them head on. In addition to helping them do that, hypnosis will also make them realize that the fear they have is illogical. Using the availability of the subconscious mind during hypnosis, this confrontation and reasoning can eliminate the fear causing the phobic reaction.

Another case of irrational fear. Subject was a middle- aged woman sent to me by a doctor. She had an abject fear that a prowler would come in through her bedroom window. As a result, she locked and bolted the second story window even in the summertime. Her house was not air conditioned. And access to the window would have had to be made by using a ladder. In spite of these facts, she had many sleepless nights.

I suggested to her doctor that I felt regression would be necessary since this fear had to have been created by some past traumatic event. He agreed.

Subject required entire session to create deep trance. Awake, she stated that she did not remember any incident which could be the cause of her fear.

During next session, regressed subject and suggested she go back slowly with my help to an earlier age and raise her right hand if she was feeling emotionally upset. Because of the possibility that these recalls might disturb her too greatly, I told her that she would not personally experience them but would be looking at them as if she were watching a movie.

Near the end of the session, she raised her right hand as the person in the movie was at the age of five. "Wait!" she cried. "That little girl! (herself) She's at the window! What's all that noise? Across the street! Dolly's house! That man's pulling Dolly out the window! He's running! Dolly's on the ground!" (Subject started to cry, then scream.)

I took her hand. "It's okay." I said calmly. "You're coming back slowly to your present age. You're in my office. Everything is fine. That memory doesn't frighten you anymore. You're calm now and will awaken slowly and comfortably when I reach the count of ten." I counted and when I reached the count of seven, I said, "When I reach the count of ten, as I told you, you will awaken and feel very relaxed. You will not be disturbed by what you were able to recall … will remember every detail of that scene you saw and be able to relate it to me calmly. I'm now counting to eight, nine, and at my next count, the count of ten, you will awaken … ten."

Recalling the incident, she related that she had a friend Dolly who lived across the street. She remembered that the police had told her father that the intruder had tried to kidnap Dolly and failed. "How could I not have remembered that?" she said.

I explained that the subconscious mind sometimes hides some memories from us if it thinks we shouldn't remember them. I could give her no explanation why that was the case here. But I did explain that it probably created the irrational fear she was experiencing.

I put her back in a trance. I said, "Tonight you will sleep with the window open and enjoy the fresh air. (It was July.) You know that the fear you had before is completely unfounded and only the result of a childhood event which didn't endanger you in any way. You will enjoy the feeling so much that you will stay awake for thirty minutes, breathing in that wonderful fresh air. Then you will sleep soundly and safely and never again be bothered by thoughts of an intruder entering your window."

Management of Pain. Pain is an electrochemical signal from the brain usually indicating something is wrong with bodily functions. It should not be ignored, and it is dangerous to continually mask it. Pain killers and hypnosis can often lessen the pain, but give temporary relief and should not be continued without an effort to correct the cause.

Tenseness of the muscles and a negative mind are known to increase the severity of pain. A positive attitude, relaxation and a proper exercise program are known to reduce pain. Relaxation also increases the amount of oxygen in the blood and this increase is known to reduce pain levels.

Much investigation into the management of pain by therapeutic research organizations also suggest that parts of the brain control the intensity of pain.

The medical term for the management of pain by hypnosis is called *hypno-analgesia.* Surgeons who have used this therapy report significant reduction in the ratings of pain, amount of sedation required, lesser loss of blood, elimination of nausea and vomiting and a shorter length of hospital stay. An additional benefit— reduction in medical and hospital expenses.

After receiving a referral from a person's doctor, a hypnotist can begin sessions to help lessen the effect of subject's pain. The subconscious mind can be addressed as follows: "Your doctor is helping manage your pain with drugs and also by prescribing procedures to discover and remedy its cause. Meanwhile, your subconscious mind can also help. You know, the tenseness of your muscles increases the severity of pain. The attitude you have toward your pain can also effect what you feel. I know it's difficult not to feel down and be negative, but a positive attitude will help to ease the pain. Let's have your mind and body help you to feel better.

"I want you to direct your mind to the area of your body that hurts. That's good. Feel your mind directing the muscles around that area to fall into relaxation. More and more as you think about that area. (Repeat last two sentences twice.) As you go deeper into relaxation, that area feels warmer and the pain seems to slide away. Away it goes. The warmth eases it away.

"Now, I want you to do just what I've suggested with your subconscious mind whenever your pain makes you feel uncomfortable.

"Easing your pain with relaxation will make you feel more positive that the medical procedures your doctor is prescribing will help to minimize your pain even more. And that positive attitude will also allow your brain to release pain killing and healing chemicals that promote healing.

"Let your subconscious help you. Let it help you to feel positive about your progress toward a cure. Let it direct you to relax completely. You are convinced that your ability to relax, your positive attitude and the release of chemicals from your brain will help you live more comfortably with your pain."

All of the preceding suggestions should be given slowly and with conviction and repeated several times. Repetition during a hypnotic trance is vitally important.

Addictions. When we think of addiction, we usually are referring to someone who is addicted to drugs or alcohol. But I think a smoker is addicted. I think anyone who drinks eight cokes a day is addicted. You get the idea. A person who is a slave to a habit pattern that dominates his or her daily existence is an addict.

Of course, drug addiction and alcohol addiction are serious and life-threatening habits. But like any addiction, *unless the addict really wants to cast the addiction out of his or her life,* they cannot be helped—not by hypnosis or by other available systems created to help the victims. And this fact is just as true with a smoker as it is with one addicted to alcohol or drugs.

I've had experience with subjects with all three types of addictions. As pointed out earlier, a smoker often asks to be hypnotized to become a non-smoker. After a session, one of my subjects didn't have a cigarette for a week. His wife called me to report that she "caught" him sneaking a cigarette in the garage. A second session produced the same result. He called a week later saying, "Thanks, but I really don't want to quit."

I'm not saying that a person under treatment can't change his or her mind. But it's a personal decision and one that's hard to make. Statistics suggest that a drug or alcohol addict will "quit" an average of eight times before giving up the habit completely.

A young man of 22 who had been addicted to heroin since he was 15, took seven sessions before he quit for the first time. He beat the average. He quit only four times after that before entering a methadone clinic for additional treatment.

When a person really does want to break an addiction, hypnosis can offer help. Strength of resolve and determination, a wonderful release from being captive to an undesirable habit, a healthier life and better quality of life—form the framework of hypnotic suggestions which can program the subconscious mind to help the subject reject urges to continue the addiction.

Just as an example of the point I made earlier. A woman I knew from church called one evening and asked if I would see her husband. She said he was an addict. "What type of addict?" I asked. "For beer," she replied. "Beer only?" was my surprised question. "Strange, isn't it? Just beer. He really wants to quit, but he doesn't think he'd like being hypnotized," she said.

At our first meeting, he agreed to "give it a try," even though he said he didn't believe in "giving up his mind." It's always remarkable, but people who have serious doubts about hypnosis' ability to help seem to be the subjects who go into a deep trance state quickly. He was one of those people.

Surprising too was the fact that he quit drinking beer after one session. But it was evident that he had a great desire and determination to give it up. That's more than half the battle.

Migraines. Migraines can be triggered by many things—ranging from a loss of sleep, to stress, to bright lights, or by one of many unrelated things. They begin with muscular tension, resulting in intense, throbbing pain. Most medical opinions state that migraines are caused by blood vessels in the head contracting followed by a painful dilation of the terminal branches of the external carotid arteries. Other assessments indicate that they are caused by swollen blood vessels pressing on nerve endings.

Although not a correction for the cause of the migraine, hypnosis has been shown to reduce the intensity of the pain by creating relaxation in and around the affected areas. If, however, they are caused by stress or anxiety, hypnosis can help to minimize the effect of stressful environments.

Clinical studies also indicate that redistributing blood flow in the brain also lessen the intensity of pain.

As with the other cases of pain symptoms, hypnosis should be indicated only after medical investigation determines there is no underlying cause for the disorder.

Surgery. Almost without exception, we all face surgery at some point in our life, and I'd like to include some remarks about it on these pages.

Significant advances in the use of hypnosis before, during and after surgery have been made in the last decade. Many hospitals have created programs offering the option for surgical patients to undergo hypnotic treatment. These treatment programs have proved the efficacy of hypnotic suggestion in relieving anxiety before surgery, reducing surgery time, minimizing blood loss, guarding against infection, reducing pain and infection—and so important— helping the healing and recovery processes.

Sounds like a miracle program, doesn't it? It isn't. It's further proof of the amazing ability of the sub-conscious mind to help us to a healthier and happier life.

The next time you're scheduled for surgery, ask your doctor about the availability of one of these programs. Other options. See a certified hypnotherapist. He will take you through steps which will lessen your anxiety during the entire process of surgery. He will offer suggestions which will make your surgery a successful and comfortable experience.

Or, if you don't want to follow that path, learn self-hypnosis. (See my blurb on self-hypnosis.) You can help yourself to get through your surgery with less anxiety, less pain and a faster and healthier recovery.

If you're going to use self-hypnosis, remember to practice putting yourself in a deep trance before you make suggestions to your subconscious mind. Then follow these steps:

Two days before surgery . . .

Hypnotize yourself. Remind yourself that the hospital where the surgery will take place has the most technologically advanced equipment available for your operation ... that the doctor who will perform your operation has performed it successfully many times ... you will be in very capable hands. You feel very positive about a successful operation. (*Repeat this several times during the day*.)

As you are taken into surgery . . .

Feel yourself going into deep relaxation. Close your eyes and say silently, "I feel very certain that my surgery will be very successful. My mind and body will be relaxed and I direct my subconscious mind to take care of all of my bodily functions while I am under the anesthetic. It will also direct my body's immune system to keep the wound dry and infection free. It will minimize bleeding and promote healing. My mind will work in cooperation with the surgeon to make the operation a success."

In the Recovery Room . . .

(When you come out of the anesthetic, put yourself into a trance.) "I now direct my defense system to promote healing throughout my entire body. Bleeding will be at a minimum and no infection will occur. My bodily functions will return to normal as will my blood pressure. I will soon be getting hungry. The area in and around the operation will begin to heal and I imagine myself getting so well that I will be leaving the hospital soon. My body is repairing itself quickly. I feel very positive." Bring yourself out of the trance and smile; you are on your way to better health!

(Remember, you don't have to use the preceding words exactly when talking to your subconscious mind. Even if you don't feel that you achieve self-hypnosis, the preceding will achieve wonderful results!)

Obstetrics. Attending the convention of the Association to Advance Ethical Hypnosis in 1953, I was astounded to see a film showing the birth of a baby by caesarian section, performed without anesthetic while the woman was deeply hypnotized. She was in a responsive state when the surgeon removed the child from her womb and held it up for her to see.

Childbirth aided by the use of hypnosis is not new but has been used very infrequently until recently. Today, it joins the popular Lamaze method as a tool for less pain before, during and after birthing. With a growing number of expectant mothers, obstetricians have been able, with hypnosis, to shorten labor, reduce or eliminate pain medications, shorten hospital stay and deliver a healthier and less traumatized infant.

As growing proof of its efficacy, research has showed that groups of expectant mothers who have participated in a program using hypnosis, required less medication by a 3 to 1 margin, had shorter hospital stays and less incident of post-partum depression.

Generally, the programs using hypnosis include a series of sessions during which the women are tested for trance depth and taught relaxation techniques. These relaxation techniques are to be used during contractions. The women are taught to welcome contractions as a step toward the joyful arrival of their newborn.. Suggestions also are given to help eliminate fear and tension.

Those obstetricians not trained to use hypnosis, refer patients to a certified hypnotherapist, who take the expectant mother through the program. Many hypnotists stay with the patient in the delivery and recovery rooms.

My practice in obstetrics has been limited to working with expectant mothers through the first two trimesters, teaching them relaxing procedures and offering them suggestions to carry them through the rest of their term and help them through the birthing process and recovery.

Dentistry. I think some people would rather go into the hospital for surgery than go to their dentist. I've hypnotized some folks simply because they were going to have their teeth cleaned!

Dentistry is one area where relaxation can make a significant difference in the measure of pain a patient feels. A tense jaw and the expectancy of pain cause pain. Dental patients who have been hypnotized report amazement at how little discomfort they felt as the dentist worked on them. Hypnotic suggestions sometimes relaxed them so completely that the dentist often had to awaken them to continue his work.

The suggestions given are simply that the subjects, when they sit in the dentist's chair, will feel a tremendous wave of relaxation come over their body and mind. They are told that this relaxation will be so profound that the only sensation they feel will be of a slight pressure on their jaw.

If a patient is in dread fear of extraction, the "glove" anesthesia method can be used. By numbing the subject's hand while in deep trance, they will be able to transfer the numbness to their jaw at their own command. A cousin of mine had this method perfected so well that she simply rubbed her jaw and it became numb in a few seconds.

Numbing the jaw with hypnosis is a fairly simple procedure. Only a medium trance is required for most subjects. However, I like to be sure, so I usually try to produce a deeper state. Creating "glove anesthesia" works well, but hypnotists have to remember to give instructions for removing the numbness created at the dentist's chair. A lot of folks would like to retain the ability to use it for other aches and pains, but instructions should be given that the procedure will be used for dental work at a given time.

Nail Biting.   I hypnotized a man who related that his father, brother and first cousin bit their nails. No, I'll correct that. His father stopped when he got his false teeth—but he had before then. The subject wanted to know if nail biting was hereditary! I've come across several cases where a father and son, or mother and daughter have had the habit so maybe there's something to it.

In any case, this man was a very good subject. Stopped biting his nails after the first session. He called me to say that his brother and cousin didn't want a "treatment" and would try to stop themselves.

Another case had an unusual twist. A young man, a sophomore in high school reported that his girl friend told him that biting his nails wasn't "very cool." Couldn't have that, so I suggested that every time he followed my suggestions and didn't put his hand to his mouth, he would feel very "cool." The suggestions worked except that he called in about a week and said, "I've quit biting my nails, but every time I stop and follow your suggestions, I feel cold!" The literal subconscious!

In both these nail biting cases, a substitute action or "anchor" was used for every time the subjects consciously or unconsciously went to bite their nails. My favorite which seems to work every time is: "When your hand, left or right, lifts toward your mouth, the middle finger of that hand will go directly to your ear and put it in your ear lightly. The urge to bite your nails will pass, your finger will drop and you will recognize that you don't want to bite your nails. Every day you will notice that your nails are growing and be proud."

Memory. It's easy to understand how hypnosis is an excellent tool when trying to dredge up the forgotten memory of a past event. As the storehouse of every action and thought we've had in our lives, of every event we've witnessed, our subconscious mind has its memory tucked away somewhere. As the "shadow knows," so does our subconscious mind.

It helps to remember another difference in our conscious and subconscious minds. With our conscious or objective mind, a memory is a recollection and can be flawed; with our subconscious or subjective mind, the memory is absolute and near perfect.

Can't remember where you "hid" a ring? "Lost" an important paper? It's such a surprise when a hypnotized subject smiles and exclaims, "I know where it is!" Not only remembers but recites many details—what day of the week it was and what they were doing before and after they hid or lost the article in question.

Naturally, when something very important happens in our lives whether it be positive or traumatic, it makes a deep impression on our brain and becomes a memory which we will remember for a long time. Conversely, what we had for breakfast two weeks ago is a memory which fades quickly.

I like to think that the impressions we receive create a cavity in our brain, deep or shallow depending

...ce of the impression. The "sands of ... as I call them, fill in those cavities over time. ...nportant memories or cavities fill in quickly and are gone. We no longer remember most of everyday happenings. But if we had an automobile accident one Tuesday afternoon, and were seriously hurt, a deep cavity is created and the sands of memory will take a very long time to fill in that cavity.

Speaking of a traumatic memory, I had an interesting case a few years back having to do with, of all things, a UFO sighting. At the time, I belonged to the Pennsylvania Association for the Study of the Unexplained. I had, and still have, a keen interest in the paranormal, and so I joined Stan Gordan's group as an investigator. Stan, knowing I was a hypnotist, asked me to try to retrieve the memory of a man who claimed he been abducted on an alien craft.

I cautioned Stan that the man could be dreaming the entire event. I also reminded him that many similar cases were proven to be a figment of an overactive imagination. This particular man was a member of Stan's group and Stan vouched for the fact that he was a very serious investigator and questioned every piece of evidence in many reported cases of alien presence.

The subject and his wife arrived at my house the next evening. I explained to him that I wanted to test his recall of an event other than the abduction before proceeding. He chose the birth of his son in the delivery room, revealing that he had been so excited and concerned for his wife that he hadn't appreciated the wonder of the important event. In a deep trance, I regressed him back to the birth day and had him slowly experience the entire procedure. Both he and his wife were in tears as he described what he saw and experienced. Before awakening him, I instructed his subconscious mind that, in the future, his mind would not allow him to describe any event which did not actually happen.

Awake still, he explained that he and a friend had taken to spending some nights on a hill where residents had reported seeing strange lights over the nearby woods. On this particular night, he and his friend made themselves a light snack and parked on top of the hill. They had, he said, a clear view of the surrounding area.

I again put him into a deep trance and reminded him that his subconscious mind would not allow him to describe anything that was not real. I also instructed him to take his time, relate his thoughts and the events as they happened. His subconscious mind would remember every word he said, every thought he had. I turned on my tape recorder.

These are his words from that tape:

(cough) "*I was thinking. This is sorta silly. Missing our sleep like this. What time is it? Lord, it's almost two o'clock. Ceil* (wife*) thinks I'm nuts.* (Silence for almost 2 minutes) *I reached over and shook Harry. He was asleep. Hey, Harry, you wanna go home? Nothin' going to happen here. People were seeing things. We didn't even eat our sandwiches. You wanna stay just ten more minutes? Okay.* (pause) *Hey look, Harry, there's a plane coming, over there, to our left. See it? Awfully low, huh.* (excited voice*) My God, Harry, that can't be a plane! Harry, what's the matter with you? Don't you see it? Wake up! He's not moving! Holy God, it's landing right over there!*

(Trembling voice) "*Damn! Where in the hell am I? That plane. That ... whatever it was. No plane. God,*

_ right. I must be on some kind of ...
_ɾe's Harry? Nowhere! What's going to happen
..ɐe? What's that noise? I'm on some kinda table.
Can't move! Can't get up! Oh, crap, someone's coming!
Who? ... That ugly son of a bitch! Those eyes! I can't
get up! What's he doing? That hurts!"

(He paused long enough for me to call his name)
"I don't remember anything else. I'm back in the car. I
can hear Harry calling my name. 'C'mon, he says. Let's
go home. I must have fallen asleep. God, it's four
fifteen! Why didn't you wake me? This is a real crock!'
He started the car. 'What about that plane? Must have
flown right over us.' As he pulled away, my sandwich
which had been above the dash board, fell on the floor. I
picked it up. It felt like a stiff board. I ... I don't know.
What happened to me?" (He started to wring his hands)

I woke him after assuring him he was okay and
would only remember the incidents of that night by
saying a trigger word ... and only when he was prepared
emotionally to relive it.

My reaction to all this? I would have to conclude
that his subconscious mind had experienced an illusion
of what he believed an abduction would be like, or he
actually had been abducted on an alien craft. I vote for
the latter.

Depression. A sensitive and somewhat "touchy" subject
where hypnosis is concerned. So, this is just a personal
opinion.

Depression in its deepest form takes the life out of
life. Literally millions of people are held in its grasp and
take many grams of expensive medicine.

Generally, depression begins its hold on a person's mental and physiological life style with a traumatic event, a negative environment, a loss of a loved one, a disturbing relationship or any one of many situations which cause sorrow and havoc with daily living. According to research, it can also run in families, can be caused by physical changes in the body, illness and stresses caused by what is felt to be excessive responsibilities.

But depression, in most cases, often does have a beginning.

I believe hypnosis can help before depression takes hold, affects the brain and requires continuing medication. It can help before depression takes hold by lessening the impact of the critical incident and creating a positive mental attitude.

Gambling. Estimates are that the availability of casinos has increased the number of people addicted to gambling tenfold. Some people can gamble for a short time and go home. Unfortunately, there are people who cannot stop and spend money they cannot afford to lose.

Why can't they stop? Is the sensation of wining so great that they keep chasing that excitement which ringing bells or the right roll of the dice brings? It's odd, but one who is addicted to gambling will name all the reasons he or she gambles and mention winning money last.

Hypnotic suggestions to help free gamblers of the addiction are built around giving them the strength to say "no" to the urge and replace it with the pleasurable sensation which turning away from it brings. The suggestions stress the benefits from giving up the undesirable habit—recovering the control of their life, and the pleasure and pride which this control brings. The hypnotist assures the subject that each time he or she says "no" to the gambling urge, the pleasure will increase and the urge will lose its hold until all interest in gambling disappears.

Addiction to gambling, like most other addictions, is difficult to beat. In one case I worked with, it took five sessions before the subject gave up the habit.

6

WHY DOES HYPNOSIS WORK?

The sixty-four thousand dollar question.

If you and I were sitting comfortably in your den, talking about this and that and I told you that when I scratched my nose, your right shoe would become very hot and would feel like it was burning your foot if you didn't take it off, what would be your reaction? Besides thinking I was crazy, I mean?

If you had been hypnotized, and were told that when you awakened, you would react quickly to the same suggestion, you would feel your shoe get hot and remove it. In the first instance, your conscious mind controlled your reaction and thought the suggestion was ridiculous because it was irrational. In the second, when you were in a hypnotic trance state, your subconscious mind had traded places with your conscious mind and reacted to the suggestion *because your subconscious mind does not have the ability to analyze between possible and impossible, logical and illogical!*

The subconscious mind can be told to create an illusion, because any one of the five senses can be "tricked" negatively or positively. After the subject is given a post-hypnotic suggestion and awakened, a person in the room can't be seen if this subject is told that he or she isn't there. This subject will not be able to hear a particular person if told that will be the case.. This subject will detect a foul odor when one isn't present. He or she will not be able to remember the name of a close personal friend. All happening as a result of a post-hypnotic suggestion.

This distinction between our two minds is why hypnosis works. The conscious mind is capable of both inductive and deductive reasoning. The subconscious mind is capable of deductive reasoning only.

The conscious mind. It's our awareness mind. It is our logical mind. It reasons, analyzes, creates, makes choices. And surprisingly, according to most scientific beliefs, it takes up only 5% of our brain mass.

The subconscious mind. A very complicated mind. It's awake every moment, from the minute we're born until we die. It cannot reason, it cannot analyze, it can't make decisions. It is a literal mind and the storehouse of everything we have experienced through our five senses. It cannot distinguish between reality and illusion.

The subconscious mind is the seat of our emotions, having stored our thoughts, feelings and memories from day one. We often react automatically to these without conscious interference because we have "trained" our subconscious mind by our decisions regarding these impulses. But if we, for example, consciously change a feeling toward a given belief or a reaction to a situation, our subconscious mind will change its reaction to that belief once our conscious mind is convinced, *and has the necessary determination,* to make the change.

As explained earlier, a hypnotized subject's conscious mind moves aside and allows access to the subconscious. Although still aware of what's going on, the conscious mind simply filters the exchange of words between the hypnotist and the subconscious mind. Unless improper verbalisms are expressed, there's no reaction from the conscious mind.

And so, that's how a desired change in behavior is helped by hypnosis. A subject expresses a desire to stop smoking or change some other unwanted behavior. They are hypnotized and the subconscious mind receives suggestions by the hypnotist. The verbalisms given to the subconscious mind cannot be rejected. They increase the desire and determination to change the behavior. These desires and determination are part of the discipline created in the subconscious.

The desire to change has already been expressed by the subject and *unless his or her conscious mind works against the suggestions given to their subconscious mind,* hypnosis will have provided the necessary ammunition to achieve the desired result. The strength of the suggestions grow as the subject cooperates and works with their subconscious mind to make the change. If the subject does not cooperate, the strength of the suggestions wanes and the change doesn't happen.

To help hypnosis be more effective, the hypnotist creates a positive image of the subject's health and life style after the unwanted habit is eliminated. He concentrates on the principal reasons the subject has for eliminating the habit For a smoker, it may be a heart problem, shortness of breath or the cost of cigarettes. For an obese person, it may also be a heart problem, diabetes or simply cosmetic.

When hypnosis helps you to give up an unwanted habit, you create a new pathway which becomes easier and easier to follow as you cooperate with the suggestions you've been given.

The important thing to remember is that each of us has a choice. Hypnosis can help to continue a desirable behavior or change an unwanted one. It can improve your mental outlook and minimize fears. It can help to lessen pain and encourage your body to heal. But it needs your help if it's to work for your benefit. It's not a magic potion or a miracle drug. And the hypnotist can't wave a magic wand and change you for the better. You've got to work with it. When you do, hypnosis can do wonderful things for you.

Why has it taken so long for the medical, therapeutic and scientific communities to recognize this?

7

DIGGING DOWN DEEP

I'm sure you all have heard about past life regression. It's when you take a hypnotized person back to a former life. Unfortunately, it's sometimes done as a parlor trick. However, past life regression has been found to be very useful in pinpointing the environment and relationships a person had during a past life or lives and studying them to ascertain what effect they may be having on present life problems and behavior.

Some people can't accept the concept that we have existed in multiple incarnations, others believe strongly that we have.

It's funny how the present day interest in past life regression was created. In 1950, a young man by the name of Morey Bernstein had just begun his practice as a hypnotist. While in a trance, his subject, Virginia Tighe, seemed to slip into an environment where she talked with an Irish accent and identified herself as a woman named Bridey Murphy.

In subsequent sessions, Bridey Murphy talked about her Irish childhood and identified many sites and areas where she had lived. Although she had never visited Ireland, many locations and buildings she mentioned while "taken back" proved to exist.

The national interest was immediate. Bernstein finally wrote a book about his experiences with Tighe. *The Search for Bridey Murphy* became required reading especially by most hypnotists.

Years later, it was discovered that Virginia Tighe had spent her early childhood in Chicago living down the street from an Irish immigrant named Bridie Murphy Corkell. But in the years before that discovery, the public's interest in past life regression grew to amazing proportions and Bridey's evident non-existence didn't quell it.

Although the use of past life regression as a therapeutic tool has increased significantly in the past decade, there still are many who have their doubts. Reasons for these doubts include a disbelief in reincarnation, the tendency of a hypnotized subject to please the hypnotist, and that many hypnotized subjects who do believe in reincarnation create a past life as a fantasy or illusion. In the hands of a hypnotist not trained to deal with all the possibility for errors in taking a subject back to past life, the past life uncovered may be an imaginary one.

I firmly believe in reincarnation and the availability of past life environments, beliefs and emotions. My religious beliefs stood in the way of this acceptance until I came face to face with Edgar Cayce, the psychic.

A religious man himself, Cayce had the unique ability to go into a self-imposed trance and mentally visit the bodies of sick people. These people did not have to be in his presence, and some of whom were half a continent away. He prescribed remedies which cured the illnesses. He didn't recall any of what he had said or prescribed while in trance.

To his surprise and utter disbelief, in one case he referred to a person's past life's relationship with a family member as the reason for a disability. This type of reference repeated itself many more times and he finally realized, and so did I as I read his life story, that we have had many past lives.

If you want to read Cayce's amazing life story, read *There is a River.*

A good example of the use of past life regression would be a case where the subject—one who believes in reincarnation and that he or she has lived a number of past lives—believes that a present life behavior or feeling may be caused by an environment in one of those past lives.

In this case I'm referring to, the subject had a unfounded dislike for a member of her family. She could not reason why she had an intense dislike for her younger sister. The hypnotist carefully regressed her back through her present life then suggested she go back through her birth and relate what she experienced. She reported being in an earlier time and different location. Asking her questions relating to her past environment and associations, it was discovered that she had been a member of a large family and lived in a large city. As the session progressed, it became obvious that she hated her mother because she had forced her to marry a man whom she didn't love and give up her true love. The marriage was one where she was abused, beaten and finally killed by her husband. In describing her mother, she said that she was a "rather skinny old hag," that had a unusual looking birthmark on the side of her right arm.

As you might suspect, so did her sister in her present life.

My involvement as a hypnotist has always been in *present life* regression. Rather than seeking help from a past life experience, present life regression seeks help from the environment and/or relationships a person has had in an earlier stage of his or her life. It is remarkable how much influence the relationships and environment we experienced in our childhoods can have on our present behavior.

Unfortunately, not all the early experiences we had as a child are positive or good. Our parents lead and guide us into life. Many times that guidance is flawed, and we are left to fight our way, a combination of our genetic heritage and environmental influencing the remainder of our life. As an adult, whatever dom-inates our personality and physical behavior is reflected from our earlier life.

Present life regression can help a person to under-stand, accept and rectify a past behavior effect on a present life or, in some cases, change an unwanted physical habit. Just becoming aware of the root of a problem, can often rectify it

Two cases illustrate the positive results from present life regression:

A stutterer. The subject, a young man of 18, stuttered badly. He lived with his grandmother. His mother was dead, his father had deserted him. His doctor, after tests, reported that there was nothing wrong systemically with his vocal mechanisms and recommended hypnosis. By the second session, subject was in a deep trance (necessary for effective regression).

At age nine, subject stuttered. At age four he did not. The particular environment which caused him to stutter existed between four and nine. To further narrow this age span, he was hypnotized again. He stuttered at age six.

Discovery phase. Under hypnosis, subject described relationship between himself and grandmother as being "terrible." Regressed to age 5, he stammered as he whined and described how "She ... she is always yelling at ... me. I'm afraid ... afraid of her."

At age 6, he stuttered badly as he described how his grandmother "always tells me I'm ba . . . bad. Hollers cause . . . cause I talk ner . . . nervous like."

Surprisingly, persons who stutter because of a negative environment and are not physically impaired, will stop stuttering with hypnotic suggestions for relaxation and a knowledge that their impairment was emotional rather than systemic. This subject, after four sessions, did not stutter when he spoke slowly. Three months later, he was able to converse normally. He stammered some when he got excited.

Sexual abuse. The subject had a story to tell. During our pre-hypnosis talk, she described the birthday party for her nine year old. She related that, at the moment her daughter cut the first slice of birthday cake, she was overwhelmed by the memory of her ninth birthday and her father tucking her into bed and fondling her improperly. She was completely confounded by the fact that she had never remembered any of her father's abuse until the moment her daughter cut her cake.

An explanation would help here. Our subconscious mind sometimes tries to protect us from traumatic memories until it feels that we are mature enough to remember them. In effect, it "calcifies" them. When her daughter observed her ninth birthday, marked by the cutting of the cake, the subject's subconscious mind used the relationship of the two incidents to release the memory of the past sexual abuse. Her mind probably felt that it was time to deal with the memory, particularly since the subject had been having severe feelings of displeasure when her husband approached her sexually.

Rightly so, the subject now felt that her childhood abuse was the reason for her negative sexual response to her husband's approaches. She sought help through hypnosis.

In many cases of early sexual abuse of women, they feel at least partly responsible for the abuse. Rarely is this true. But the trauma of discovery is the first step in putting the negative effect of the abuse in its proper perspective. It should no longer have any effect on present enjoyment of sexual experience with a mate.

Hypnotic sessions concentrate on rejecting negative responses to sexual abuse by first convincing the subject that the real and only responsible factor in the abuse was, in this case, her father. And that she had given no consent to his actions. Second, that her memory of the abuse would no longer affect her desire and enjoyment of sexual experience. Several sessions helped subject to accept these suggestions.

The subconscious mind is the storehouse of memories of all that has happened in our lives. Some are flitting, unimportant ones, soon to be forgotten. Others may make a deep impression and are forever imprinted on our minds. Some hide from us but can affect our behavior. Hypnosis can uncover them, help to understand the basis for their effect on our present life, and minimize their control over our behavior.

8

GOING INTO A HYPNOTIC TRANCE

Ever notice how youngsters, sitting in front of the television watching their favorite cartoon characters are so engrossed that they don't seem to hear when they're called? They seem to be in a trance, don't they? For that matter, so do you when your favorite soap opera or exciting who-done-it is on the same screen. The point is you are, and so is the youngster, in a light trance. Your conscious mind is practically oblivious to what else is going on around you. You're in a light hypnotic trance.

What you're experiencing is the first of three levels of hypnotic trance states. Your brain is working at about seven to fourteen cycles per second. It's called the Alpha state. Same as a light level of sleep. Surprisingly, most of the behavioral problems you might have can be addressed and helped in this light trance state. The trance which you or the youngster was experiencing as you watched television was created by your rapt attention to the action on the screen. In hypnosis, your attention, with your approval, is captured by the suggestions given by the hypnotist.

A hypnotist can use any one of countless ways to create a trance state. Almost all are intended to capture the subject's attention and lead him or her to a depth of relaxation which allows the subconscious mind to come to the fore.

I've seen a list of 38 different symptoms which define what depth of trance a subject is in, but it's very confusing to everyone except the person who made the list.

For the sake of discussion, I'd like to suggest that there are just three basic trances. No surprise ... light, medium and deep. That latter state is called somnambulism. It really means one who walks in their sleep, but hypnotists have borrowed it to indicate a very deep trance.

How can a hypnotist tell which state you are in? That list does help here. For example, when you're in a light trance, your breathing tends to be slower and deeper, your pulse rate also slower. You have partial limb catalepsy, which means you may not be able to bend your arm or move it up or down if the hypnotist suggests it. If he suggests you can't open your eyes, you will not be able to if you're in this light trance.

When you're in medium trance, your brain waves operate at 4 to 7 cycles per second. Sounds very scientific, but all it means is that you're relaxing much deeper. There's no specific way to tell when you slide from light to medium, but if the hypnotist feels that this deeper trance state will be required to achieve the desired result, there are tests, such as creating complete amnesia of an important event in the life of the subject.

In this medium trance state, the hypnotist can create both positive and negative illusions of the five senses. There are also many other "tricks" of the mind which can be created. Examples: a person in the room can be made to be invisible to the subject, a subject will not hear a given person in the room but hear others; a piece of candy will be made to taste like a lemon, and many others.

Not everyone will reach the somnambulistic state. This is Delta and the brain operates at 0 to 4 cycles per second. I have found that working with a subject through a number of sessions can deepen the trance each time to enable me to achieve many of the results possible in this somnambulistic state.

This deep state allows the hypnotist to regress the subject to an earlier age so that specific environments can be pinpointed, investigated and uncovered to enable both subject and hypnotist shed light on the cause of a behavioral problem.

I have used this present-life procedure in helping, as illustrated earlier, stutterers, sexual abuse victims, as well as those with seemingly unexplainable behaviors or various forms of addiction which may be the result of earlier life environments.

9

SELF-HYPNOSIS

There are only two people who can hypnotize you. A hypnotist and you.

When a hypnotist does it, it's called heterohypnosis. When you do it, it's *self-hypnosis,* a way you can help yourself with any problems or needs you might have. Self-hypnosis is easy to achieve but it takes practice.

We all talk to ourselves, and self-hypnosis is just that. Telling yourself what you want to accomplish. If you prefer, you can think to yourself instead, but I've found that talking out loud makes a deeper impression on the mind. To get the best results, you should be able to take yourself into deep relaxation—and this is where the practice comes in. Each time you sit in a comfortable chair (or lay on a couch), and talk yourself into a relaxed state, you'll find that you go deeper and deeper. The deeper you go the more effective the suggestions you give yourself will be.

If you don't want to take the time to practice, I'll tell you a secret. Go see your favorite hypnotist and he'll put you in a deep trance, give you a post-hypnotic trigger which will allow you to put yourself into a deep trance … and voilà … you're there in a minute!

Either way you can use your subconscious mind to improve many facets of your life, correct unwanted habits, teach yourself the self discipline you need to accomplish any change in behavior.

Supposing you're not happy with the 200 pounds you're carrying around and would like yourself much better if the scale read "175." If you are really determined to lose those 25 pounds, practice relaxing yourself many times until you feel that your subconscious mind is ready to listen. Remember, your subconscious mind will help you every time you're tempted to give in to those habits which add to your weight problem.

Maybe this will help you get started with the right verbalisms to use. I've used words such as these with a subject who needs help shedding a few pounds. I've substituted the word "my" instead of "your" in the following. You should use them in self-hypnosis.

(*After you are in a trance state*) "My subconscious mind is going to give me all the necessary desire, determination and discipline needed to help me lose the pounds I want to lose. I now have an image of myself as I will look after I lose those pounds and that image will appear before me every time I am tempted to eat the wrong foods, eat too much or eat between meals." (*Repeat the above, speaking slowly and with emphasis and picture yourself as you want to look.*)

"I will eat three meals a day but will limit myself to smaller portions and eat only those foods I know will help me maintain or lose weight." (*If you're still working*: "I will eat a salad with a few crackers or have a piece of fish for lunch. No snack in the afternoon.")

"I will prepare a regular dinner for my family (or myself) but I will have only smaller portions for myself. I will not have snacks during the evening, will not eat before I retire, knowing that taking food to bed with me will be harmful in my effort to lose weight. My subconscious mind will help me to be satisfied with the food I've eaten and feel pleased with my day.

"Many times a day the image of my new self will remind me of my determination to lose those 25 pounds." (*Repeat this paragraph again*)

"Tonight when I go to sleep my subconscious mind will reinforce these suggestions I've given myself, strengthening them. As I drift off to sleep, I will see myself as a slimmer person, very pleased with how I will look as I keep up my program of eating properly. I will exercise every day to help me keep my body firm."

If you're a smoker, see Chapter 5. You can tailor your verbalisms to suit your situation.

Remember, check with your doctor if you have a "nagging" problem which continues to worry you and has been bothering you for an unusually long time.

In teaching classes on self-hypnosis, I remind members of the class that self-hypnosis can help in an unlimited number of ways. (See my list in Chapter 3) It will give you the stamina and the courage you need to achieve the results you desire. And remember, practice until you can create a state of relaxation that will open your subconscious mind to positive suggestions.

10

WHAT ABOUT MEDITATION?

Meditation has been practiced for many centuries by many of the Eastern religions. Yoga classes include many sessions devoted to meditation. As is the case with hypnosis, the practice of meditating has been growing in popularity.

There are similarities between the two. The major difference, in my opinion, is that hypnosis goes beyond the state of relaxation and establishes a connection with a person's subconscious mind, accomplishing improvements and corrections in personal behavior. When one meditates, the mind is released and finds its own way to various arenas of thought.

Most types of meditation use deep breathing techniques to induce relaxation. The result is a focusing of attention on the moment. Some use a mantra—a word, a sound to help eliminate outside interference with thoughts.. Others use music.

Many people attending my classes practice meditation. They become excellent subjects for hypnosis because of their experience with relaxation techniques. I always encourage them to continue. It's a good habit to practice.

11

HYPNOSIS IN POLICE WORK

It's called forensic hypnosis, and the fight has been going on for decades!

The combatants? The police departments who regularly use hypnosis to enhance memory recall of witnesses and victims in criminal cases and the courts who rule against the acceptance of information obtained by hypnosis.

There are records of hypnosis use as a forensic tool which go back almost a century, but since the 1970s, there has been an increased use of hypnosis by many police enforcement agencies. They have personnel trained as hypnotists who can uncover memories of key witnesses to a crime. One of the most successful agencies in this effort has been the Los Angeles Police Department. One statistic reported by this agency states that additional information obtained through hypnosis helped crime solving in 81% of the cases in which it was used. This information led investigators to arm themselves with sufficient evidence to lead to convictions.

The investigators trained in the use of forensic hypnosis must exercise extreme care in questioning witnesses. Remembering that hypnotic subjects are in a suggestible state, the investigator must not lead the witness toward a desired result. The investigator would ask, "Where were you on the night of _____?" and not, "Were you on the corner of (such and such) on the night of _____ ?" "Why were you there?" Plus other questions or statements allowing the witness to describe what he or she saw or experienced.

The information obtained by forensic hypnosis can serve a number of purposes. It can add to and/or qualify the evidence already obtained by arresting officers; it can help to obtain confessions from the accused; it can help prosecuting attorneys in preparing their case; if the court allows, the evidence obtained during hypnosis can be presented in court.

The public may not be aware of it, but forensic hypnosis has been used in quite a few famous cases. Although information obtained was not always presented in court, it led to the arrest and conviction of such criminals as the Boston Strangler. In this case, a witness identified Ted Bundy as the driver of a van in which one of his victims was riding. In another, Sam Sheppard was exonerated in the killing of his wife when he was able under hypnosis to describe the killer. This case later became the basis for the movie *The Fugitive*.

In a well-publicized case, when a school bus driver and 45 children were abducted and buried alive, the driver was able to escape and later, under hypnosis, remembered the license plate number of the abductor's vehicle.

In 1988, The Supreme Court ruled that hypnosis was an acceptable interviewing technique to obtain information from witnesses and victims of crimes. It didn't state that this information was acceptable in court. Some states put hypnosis in the same class as polygraph testing. A majority of states legislate against its acceptance as a procedure for uncovering legally acceptable information.

It's the same old story. Officials who know little about hypnosis are hesitant to allow information recovered from conscious memory loss as actual and reliable evidence.

12

SLEEP/TALK

During World War II, the military experimented with a procedure I now call Sleep/Talk. They saw the necessity of training some military personnel to understand and speak Japanese. They divided a class into two groups, teaching the Japanese language to both during daytime classes but using tapes with the control group at night. After this group was asleep, tapes were placed under their pillows. These tapes reinforced the teaching that they had been given during the day, The results were as was hoped. The control group learned the language much faster and, surprisingly, spoke Japanese without an American accent.

The use of hypnosis during sleep isn't new and recorded instruments have been available for many years. What intrigued me was its possible use with very young children who hadn't reached the age where these instruments and the use of hypnosis would be effective … for such behaviors as bed wetting, thumb sucking or personal relationships with family members.

The idea struck me one night when my wife and I were visiting a friend's house.

Our friend had three sons, one of whom was 14 and still wet the bed. He and I had a great rapport, having talked sports and school work many times. I was surprised when his mother told me of this unwanted habit. It was 11 o'clock when she told me this and the boy had been asleep for over an hour. I asked if I could "try something." Like many of our friends, she wasn't aware that I practiced hypnotism.

I went up to his room, sat by his bed, and quietly spoke his name. I introduced myself and began talking in a low voice. I didn't have to hypnotize him because his subconscious mind was already available to me. My suggestions were simply that whenever he would feel the urge to urinate, he would awaken slowly and recognize the urge. He would then have a great desire to get up and go to the bathroom. I repeated these instructions several times.

His mother's first question was, "What did you do?' "I gave him a few suggestions," I replied. "About what?" she asked. "Just to help him break his habit of wetting the bed," I said. My wife interrupted at this point. "Bill's a hypnotist. He just gave your son some suggestions. Maybe you won't have to change the bed sheet tomorrow morning."

She didn't. And she called me and gave me the devil because I hadn't done it years before.

It got me to wondering. Even though the friend's son was 14, why couldn't suggestions be given to little ones under the age when hypnosis usually isn't recommended or effective because of a limited attention span and help eliminate unwanted habits? That question got me started with Sleep/Talk.

Sleep/Talk is based on the same principles used in hypnosis *but is not hypnosis.* A child in deep sleep is as relaxed as a hypnotic subject in a deep trance. As a little child sleeps, their conscious mind sleeps but their sub-conscious mind is open to positive suggestions. It hears these suggestions and their effect can create a desire to achieve what is suggested.

Sleep/Talk is an innovative procedure for parents to help their child end bed wetting, thumb sucking, nail biting or other undesirable habits. It can also be used to improve conduct and control actions.

If you were a parent using Sleep/Talk, these steps would be followed:

1. Sit beside the bed as close to the child as possible.
2. Make sure the child is asleep by whispering his or her name. If he or she stirs, wait a moment and repeat name.
3. Make light contact with the child by touching a hand or arm, being sure not to exert too much pressure.
4. Begin by speaking the child's name and introducing yourself. "Kevin, this is Mommy. I want you to stay asleep as I talk to you about something very important to both of us." If the child awakens, wait a few moments and begin again.

Supposing "Kevin," aged five, wets the bed. Here is a sample script a mother could use in talking to him: (*Speak slowly*)

"Kevin, you are getting to be such a big boy. Daddy and I are so proud of you. It's such a wonderful joy for us to see you getting older and becoming a young man." (*Here cite some example of progress he has made lately—taking his own bath, dressing himself, etc.*)

"You know, Kevin, as you grow older, you start to do the things older children do. Why, it won't be long before you start elementary school and learn many new and interesting things—you'll even learn to read and write just like mommy and daddy (and siblings if appropriate).

"Growing up will be so much fun for you. You'll be able to do the things you've seen older boys and girls do. That's what growing up really is—not doing the things you did as a baby and doing more grown-up things. First thing you know, Kevin, you'll be a grown-up person.

"It may seem funny to you, Kevin, but mommy and daddy were your age a long time ago. And we did the things you've done—we ate baby food and slept in a crib too. But you don't do those things anymore because you're becoming a big boy and have stopped those baby habits.

"Mommy knows that you have been having a little trouble getting rid of one of those habits that many young children have. And that's wetting the bed. It's nothing to worry about, because we know that real soon you'll stop doing it. But I'd like to give you a little help so you can stop it right now. You see, Kevin, when you wet the bed it's just that you don't wake up completely and get up and go to the bathroom—or maybe you feel that it's just not worth the trouble. To get up.

"I know you want very much to stop wetting the bed, so here's what's going to happen.

(Slowly and with emphasis*)* *"From now on, when you have to go, you will wake up and have a great desire to get up and go to the bathroom. You will be so proud of yourself as you get up because you know that's what big boys do. Let me tell you again. Your mind and body will tell you when you have to go and you will wake up and realize that going to the bathroom is just what big boys do at night when they have to go. And getting up then will make you feel so proud. And you know what? Mommy and Daddy will be so proud of you too!"*

If one night's attention doesn't produce the desired result, the procedure is repeated. A child's subconscious probably will not respond to suggestions as soon as an adult mind. And their bladder control has to be trained. The verbalisms should be repeated for any many nights as it takes to eliminate the habit pattern.

Thumb sucking is an instinctive behavior. Tests have shown that a baby may even suck its thumb in the womb. It's a habit which brings comfort and pleasure to a baby and is instinctive because of the baby's desire to breast feed. It is often a daytime habit as well.

Sleep/Talk will help to eliminate the thumb sucking habit. The same verbalisms used for bed wetting with obvious changes should be used. A mother I encouraged to use Sleep/Talk for her thumb-sucking son, gently pulled his thumb from his mouth as she talked to him. She then said, "See, David, you sleep just as comfortably without your thumb in your mouth." She repeated this suggestion for a number of nights.

For the first several nights, he returned his thumb to his mouth. Four nights later, as she tucked him in, he looked up at her and said, "I don't think I'll need my thumb tonight, Mommy."

As children grow older, they can be helped in many ways with Sleep/Talk: with school work, in areas of behavior, relationships with parents, siblings and school mates. It's amazing how it can help with performance in sports activity. I'd like to take credit for a number of home runs in Little League play, but Sleep/Talk has made sluggers out of many a very backward batter. Here's where the dad is the talker.

With older children I've hypnotized for various behavior problems, Sleep/Talk gives a parent a way to continue the suggestions after my hypnotic sessions have been concluded. One case comes to mind.

This young man was an excellent Little Leaguer. He was a member of a select traveling team that had been put together from a number of teams. He was doing fine, batting over .500 until he got hit with a pitch. His average dropped dramatically. He began stepping back as the pitcher threw the ball—a habit called "stepping in the bucket."

After a hypnotic session, he again returned to is old form of smacking the ball around—until he got hit with a pitch again. Hypnosis again. Excellent batter again. His father called me. Guess what. This was getting very expensive for him.

I offered a solution. I instructed the father to Sleep/Talk his son, using the same suggestions I had used during our hypnosis sessions. They worked as well, the father reported.

If you're a parent, why not use Sleep/Talk with your children? Are they backward, not sure of themselves? Do they need help performing in school sports? Getting more interested in school work? Need help getting along with family members? You don't have to be a psychologist to help them. Use common sense suggestions. They work.

We have a lot of fun during classes when we discuss Sleep/Talk. Many of the women want to know if they could Sleep/Talk their husbands into making the beds and washing the dishes. As far as I know, my wife hasn't Sleep/Talked me—yet!

13

MOTIVATION

There is a whole laundry list of goals for which people need and want to be motivated.

For children it can be better performance in school, in sports, in behavior, in social graces and many others. (More often than not, it's the parents who want the child to be motivated.)

For adults, the goal can be any one of a hundred or more. It can include: becoming a better person, more successful in business, improved marriage and personal relationships, healthier habits, achieving greater self-esteem, overcoming procrastination, being successful in sports (golf especially!), achieving social status, becoming a better parent. Did I miss any? It really doesn't matter. The hypnotic suggestions which help to motivate follow the same basic pattern for each.

Regardless of what a person's need for motivation is, suggestions to the subconscious mind have proved to be excellent motivators. Excellent because they move people into high gear towards a goal that seems to have eluded them.

The first thing a person needs is determination. Second is a reachable goal. Third is a strong commitment to work untiringly toward that goal. Quite frankly, I tell subjects that it's a choice they have to make and remind them that the subconscious mind is a strong motivator as long as they listen and follow the suggestions given it.

During the first hypnotic session, we discuss the goal which the subject wants to reach, what obstacles might be in the path of reaching it, and how determined they are to make the change a permanent part of their life style. During this initial session, I like to determine the subject's trance depth. In successive sessions, suggestions are given to create what I call a "fist-clenching" determination to achieve the goal. This strong determination is, I believe, the most important motivator in reaching the desired goal.

In my experience, it usually takes three or four sessions to help people to completely escape the old habits and beliefs which have stood in the way of achieving a goal. When they are successful, they create one of the most rewarding experiences a person can have—the pleasure and pride that goes with achieving a goal they felt was unreachable.

14

WHAT ABOUT HYPNOSIS
AND HEALING?

Thirty years ago, a hypnotist who expressed an opinion about the possibility of healing through hypnosis would have been not only a brave soul but one who would have raised a few eyebrows. Using the mind and body's own capability to heal? Using the subconscious mind to ease the pain of cancer patients, of expectant mothers' contractions, of surgery patients during and after surgery? And accomplishing these wonderful results simply by directing the remarkable subconscious mind to harness the body's healing forces? I wasn't one of the brave souls. But I am now and have been for a long time.

Most certified hypnotists, myself included, have always been convinced of the subconscious mind's capability to work wonders by helping subjects to correct or eliminate behavioral problems. And we discovered that our suggestions to hypnotized subjects were also able to mentally address their areas of bodily pain and relax them so the pain was lessened.

For many years, experienced, certified hypnotists have believed that suggestions to the subconscious mind can heal broken bones more quickly, lessen pain and reduce the medications required, help doctors and patients attack cancer cells and causes of debilitating diseases.

Why do we believe this? Because we've found that our subconscious mind, in addition to running all of our autonomous systems, is capable of facilitating blood flow, directing and strengthening our immune system, producing healing hormones and helping us to a shorter recovery time from wounds and surgery.

Do you happen to remember the first time you cut your finger? If you were just a child, your mother probably soothed you, maybe kissed your finger and put a band-aide on it. In the meantime, your subconscious mind rushed antibodies and white blood cells to the area to fight infection and start the healing process. It was automatic. It was your immune system at work.

This immune system is part of our biological structure, and is controlled by our subconscious mind. It distinguishes negative organisms from healthy cells and has the ability to direct an attack against invaders such as bacteria, viruses and cancer cells. Hypnotic suggestions concentrate the capability of the subconscious mind to attack these negative forces.

The common denominator of treatment for healing procedures is relaxation, best achieved by hypnosis. Suggestions create a positive attitude, determination, desire and a belief that the subconscious mind has the capability to heal.

After prescription by a doctor, I like to schedule a series of sessions to work with subjects to establish their achievable depth of trance, their determination to help themselves and belief that they can be helped, followed by sessions which deal with the specific disorder in question. During these latter sessions, I have found that using imagery is an excellent tool in directing the subconscious mind's immune system to fight the disorder. I often liken their immune system as a troop of soldiers attacking and killing the "bad" disease-causing cells—or a violent whirlwind blowing them down into a bottomless pit—or any symbolic type of attack selected by the subject.

Any attempt to help a subject to minimize pain through hypnotic relaxation should always recognize that pain is a warning signal from the body that an organic disorder probably exists.

Slowly but surely, the medical and therapeutic professionals have come to accept the fact that healing, both physical and mental, often requires more than medicine and simple therapeutic consultations.

Can you imagine how we hypnotists feel now that hypnotism is finally getting the recognition it has deserved for many years? There's still a way to go, but we are beginning to win the battle.

15

A CHANCE OF A GHOST

What would the word "ghost" be doing in a book about hypnosis?

In this case, it manages to be part of a story about a long-time friend. He (we'll call him Ed) came to visit one evening asking to be hypnotized. "I'd like to remember some details I can't recall about some strange things that have happened in our house the last couple of weeks." He looked at me rather sheepishly and added, "We've got a ghost in one of our bedrooms."

He explained. "As you know, Ann and I live in an old house. One part is over two hundred years old. Other section is only one hundred. Our girls (one baby sleeps in a crib, the older one is five) sleep in a bedroom in the older section. Ten days ago, Tuesday it was, Ann asked me to check the girls in this back bedroom." He sighed and said, "When I walked in the room, there was this real warm feeling that hit me. I stepped in further and checked the bed and the little crib. Everything was fine. Duff," he said," you gotta believe me. There was this … person, an older woman, I think, sitting in the rocking chair in the corner." He looked at me with raised eyebrows and said, "She was just sitting there. She wasn't … whole, I mean … solid. Just sorta transparent like."

"What did you do then?" I asked smiling.

"I stood there," he said, ignoring my apparent amusement. "The girls seemed okay, so I got the hell out of there"

It seemed that Ed's wife had seen the same apparition several times and wanted his reaction and explanation. Their description of the "lady" wasn't exactly the same.

"Can you hypnotize me and have me remember all that I saw … and felt?"

"Sure, Ed," I replied. "But how's that going to help?"

"It will maybe let me know what she wants and why's she there."

I thought for a moment. "She probably used to live in your house and she is just returning for a visit"

"Why?" Ed asked.

"I don't know. She could have been gone a long time ago. Anyhow, if you want to relive that scene in the room, let me hypnotize you. Maybe you'll see something you don't remember now and it will help."

After fighting relaxation for a while, Ed dropped into a deep trance. I regressed him back to the night in question and walked him down the hall to the girl's room. I reminded him that he would be calm as he observed every detail of his next five minutes in the room.

What he remembered didn't help much. He did describe the woman a little better than he had reported earlier. "She had on a long black dress with a white collar. Couldn't see her shoes. But she was smiling. And rocking in the chair!" He squirmed. "Seemed friendly. I felt she was sorta watching over them!"

I told him to walk out of the room and I awakened him slowly.

"Well?" he asked.

"Nothing much," I replied. "Not much help. But maybe I can find out who she is."

"You can?"

"Maybe," I said. "Just maybe."

Just to make a long ghost story shorter, here's what I did to get the solution to Ed and Ann's problem.

I know a clairvoyant in Ohio with whom I had worked on a few other similar cases And I contacted her. Only facts she wanted were Ed's address, the girl's ages, and what Ed and Ann saw. "I'll contact you in about a week," she promised me.

If you aren't aware of how clairvoyants work, this will be rather unbelievable to you, but my clairvoyant friend called me about ten days later. This is what she told me. Don't ask me how she knew.

"Her name is Sophie. You're right, she did live in that section of the house—before an addition was built. This happened more than a hundred and fifty years ago (that would put it in the early 1800s or late 1700s) and there still were a few tribes of uncivilized Indians in the area. They stole her baby one night when her husband John was hunting. She has spent all these years looking for her baby and refuses to go on until she finds her.

When they put their young ones in that room, she was convinced their young one was her baby. She doesn't know any better because her emotions are so high and her desire to find her baby has been her only reason for existing."

"What can I do to help them ... help Sophie?"

"You must go to that room and tell her the truth. That her baby has gone through the light and is probably in the light and awaiting her. Tell her that. Tell her that she will find her baby by turning to the light and walking into it. Her friends and her husband will receive her and take her to her child."

"Should I be the one to do this?" I asked.

"You are more in tune," she said. Thanks, I said to myself.

Seeing a ghost won't be my first time, but I never had the nerve to try talking to one. I told Ed and Ann what had to be done and they agreed. Easy for them to say!

It should have been a cold winter's night with the wind howling, but it was summer and pleasant when I sat in the room and waited for Sophie. Every once in a while, with only the light from the hallway allowing me to make out the rocking chair and two children in their beds, I could see a wisp of something sitting there. Wasn't really sure.

About fifteen minutes after I entered the room, some semblance of Sophie appeared. I gave my speech—explaining what the clairvoyant had told me. I waited. Nothing. I repeated my message. The room seemed (maybe it was my imagination) to get cold ... or normal. There was a disturbance in the corner where the rocking chair was. As I watched, my hair bristling, a soft flash left the room through the outside wall. The room seemed to get warmer immediately. Sophie was gone.

End of story. Sophie never appeared again. Ed and Ann were happy, for a while. Other ghosts appeared in their old basement. "You talk to them," I told them.

16

MY LAST WORDS

Every certified hypnotist has faced many obstacles as
he or she has tried to convince others of the merits and
place that hypnosis should play in helping professionals
and referred subjects create a better and healthier life
style.

Depending on when the hypnotist began practicing,
the obstacles have been many or fewer. I happened, as I
said earlier, to run across many raised eyebrows when I
offered help for a behavioral problem to a friend or to a
subject who had been referred to me. That was back in
the 1950s, before Erickson, before the approval of
hypnosis as an acceptable adjunct to medical treatment
by the American and British Medical Associations. Only
my immediate family, not even my close relatives, knew
that I practiced hypnosis. For that matter, some of the
latter still don't.

Far too often, I have been disappointed and frustrated by the poor reception given hypnosis by professionals and medical facilities. It is also very disturbing to pick up a newspaper and ready a lengthy article about "mind-body" training, search the pages, read about "deep breathing" and "relaxation," plus yoga, Reiki and other treatments that "help the mind, body and spirit work together in the healing process" … and read not one word about hypnosis.

More disturbing is the fact that every one of the techniques mentioned is rooted in the same principles and practices of hypnosis that hypnotists have been following every time they create a trance state.

Many hospitals are also establishing what they often refer to as "mind-body" clinics. Nurses and other "care personnel" are being trained, not by hypnotists or hypnosis organizations, but by a growing number of health institutes. Hypnosis is not on their agenda. Some of these hospitals are also staffing volunteers who are Reiki masters (although some are also hypnotists) and call them in to help patients in need of pain control, anxiety and healing.

Why isn't hypnosis given the same status?

Perhaps we have only ourselves to blame.

In my early days as a hypnotist, it was a tough job convincing people who asked if hypnosis could help them with a behavioral problem. I found that hypnosis was scoffed at by medical and therapeutic professionals. A number of doctors, especially psychiatrists, refused to see me. I was very dismayed when one doctor described me as a "quack, playing around with people's minds."

I felt like an apostle trying to sell a faith-healing process.

I wasn't much comforted by the realization that hypnosis had, many times in its history, fallen to periods of disinterest. Was it going to happen again? There are a few people and organizations to thank that it didn't happen—a few hypnotists who had the unwavering faith in the benefits which hypnosis could bring to the medical and therapeutic professions. And give credit also to the stage hypnotist, even though this entertainment side of hypnotism didn't help the serious aspects of the art, it kept interest in hypnosis alive.

So, once again, hypnosis is regaining its acceptance as a procedure to help medical and therapeutic professionals help people. But, in spite of the fact that hypnosis is a completely safe procedure, prescriptions for drugs which conceivably could endanger the health and well-being of individuals are being written every day. Pharmacological companies are spending millions developing and promoting these drugs whose possible side effects can be alarming.

Organizations such as the National Guild of Hypnotists and satellite groups such as my local Hypnotism Society of Pennsylvania have taken up the mantle and are encouraging their members to become apostles too. These members have to take every opportunity to educate both the lay person and professionals as to where hypnosis fits as an adjunct to medical and therapeutic treatments.

I hope what you have read here gives you a better understanding of how hypnosis may be able to help you to a better and healthier life style. Do you or a member of your family have a behavior problem? Hypnosis can help. It can help in so many ways, Ask your doctor how he feels about hypnosis as a help with a treatment you are currently undergoing or will need.

There are many certified hypnotists who can help. The National Guild of Hypnotists can refer you to satellite organizations in your area. They can put you in touch with an experienced certified practitioner. Head-quartered in Merrimack, New Hampshire, they can be reached at 603-429-9438. Here in Western Pennsylvania, the Hypnotism Society of Pennsylvania has many members and will be happy to put you in touch with a certified hypnotist. Reach them on their website on Facebook at "Hypnotism Society of Pennsylvania."

Note: Many communities and professional organizations welcome speakers who cover interesting topics. Many certified hypnotists would like to reach out to these groups. If your church or social group or professional organization would like one of the members of the Society to make a presentation about hypnosis and how it helps promote a better and healthier life, get in touch with either one of these groups.

ABOUT THE AUTHOR

Bill Duffy, is a native of Pittsburgh, Pennsylvania and lives there with his wife Mary. They have six children, 15 grandchildren and 16 great-grandchildren (and counting). When asked about his extended family, Bill reports that they are trying to populate the earth.

He served three and a half years in the military. He was in the army's artillery branch until he transferred to the public relations service in the Philippines and covered the war crime trails of Japanese Generals Yamashita and Homma as an army correspondent.

His interest and training in hypnosis began at Duquesne University, under the tutelage of his psychology professor. After his military service, he resumed his studies under a hypnotist who had served in military hospitals as a medical hypnotist.

His practice is now limited to hypnotizing subjects referred by doctors and referrals by former subjects, teaching classes in hypnosis and his innovative Sleep/ Talk procedure and lecturing to various groups.

Bill Duffy is a certified member of the National Guild of Hypnotists and the Hypnotism Society of Pennsylvania. His e-mail: glduf3@yahoo.com.